ISBN:

This is a book about processing
and grief. Provide knowledge.
And my experience to be able
to help people. Reading studies.
*Can we ourselves do something
trying to avoid Parkinson's? Yes.
NOT only if someone gets it.

It is primarily a book for the
relatives with Parkinson's
disease.
There are many of us who are
affected in different ways.

This is my way of dealing with
grief, that mom is ill.
It feels like a diary for me also.
And some want to talk, and
others just want to be quiet.

I'm trying to understand
Parkinson's disease.
I read many studies from
scientists.
I am not a doctor or nurse.
My thought's as I understand in
a very simple way:
Let's call it: Parkinson's
"Dots forming Clusters"
They try to "eat" their way into
the brain cells.
That kills the substance
dopamine.
The one that makes you feel joy.

And all the horrible symptoms
that come with it. Memory loss,
everything according to time
passes. Stress can worsen and
poor sleep.

Healthy Brain cells & Sick Brain cells

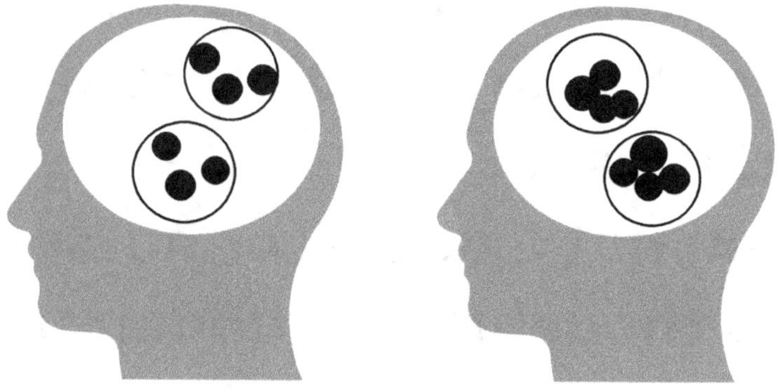

BLACK DOTS = Protein

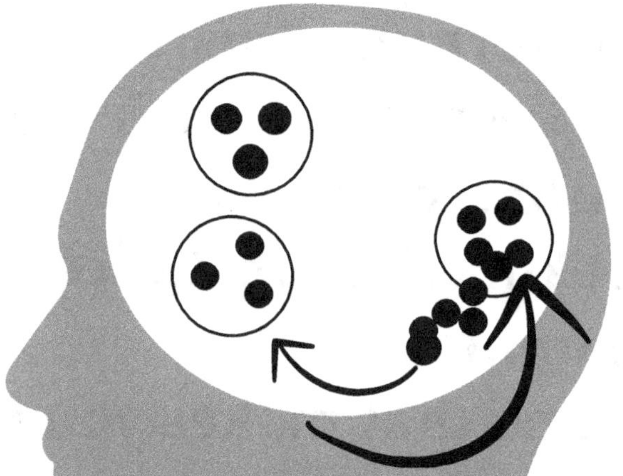

Special Protein = "Parkinson", that has become a cluster. Wanting to get into a healthy brain cell.

Some studies from doctors and research in the United States. They found that blood vessels damage, affect very much. And it can start to affect the memory, if you do not get enough good blood flow to the brain.
By having a good sleep, we can try to "avoid" it.
The brain works at night too. Trying to repair the brain.
Eating healthy food, omega 3, magnesium, vitamin B.
And move. They see that the stomach, and the connection to the incredibly many blood vessels in the brain. Are of great importance.

Research shows that:
Blueberries contain antioxidants. And helps the brain produce neurotransmitter.
Thus protecting your brain, from oxidative stress and inflammation. Blueberries can make new healthy brain cells. And Parkinson's disease " eats up " healthy brain cells slowly.
More healthy food for the brain:
Fatty fish, Eggs, Broccoli, Oranges, Coffee, Nuts, Dark chocolate 80%
Pumpkin seeds, Turmeric, Vitamins and minerals.

But how can you detect it?
How long? Scientists have
been trying to figure that out.
But it's very different.
Some say two years.

I don't know, when mom might
have started to
have small symptoms.
It's many years.
It's a creeping disease.
But I remembered her saying:
-I think I lost my sense of smell.
It is a very weak and a
slow process.

A study from a man in the
United States, who got
Parkinson's he said:

Year 2000 : His sense of smell deteriorated.

Year 2000 : He got tremor in his right hand.

Year 2004 : Tremor in right hand and leg. And stopped swinging his arm as he walked.
Also, pill-rolling tremor.
That is an early sign with Parkinson's disease.

He started to write very small. Numbers, and short term memory.
Eat slowly.
Cogwheel Rigidity.

Year 2013 : He started to get tremor on both sides.
He did exercise weight muscle lifting.
And stretching. He goes on a very strict diet. Keto diet.

He exercises in the mornings.
He drinks only coffee at the morning with butter.
And he avoids carbs.
He eats healthy green salad.
He feels better in the symptom.

*Eat plenty of protein - but not together with levodopa medications,
at the same time.

Parkinson's is like a slow
torture. In many different ways.
Often many years.
I don't think my mom has much
time left.

She is a real fighter.

She takes about 12 tablets a day,
That affects her body and brain.
In a good and a bad way.

I miss her joy of life.
All conversations about
everything between
"sky and sea".

It has not been easy for her.
But we fight together.

I remember one day, when I
came to visited
her. I helped her with her
socks. I said something she
thought was funny.
It made me realize, how long
ago, I heard her laugh.

It was a lovely feeling but
still so sad.
Parkinson's disease,
all dopamine disappears.
What makes you feel happy.
And you start shaking,
you can't walk, eat, swallow.
All organ fade away slowly.
You can hallucinate, and it is
hard to understand things.

I was going to seek help from
the church. But I feel this is a
good way for me to process.

Everyone grieves in different
ways. And nothing is wrong.
Writing helps many.
And I need to feel good,
to be able to help my mom.
But I feel guilty when I'm not
with her.
You don't die of your
Parkinson's it is said that.
It's the symptoms.

My mom has all the
symptoms now.
It hurts body and mind to see
her suffer.

Some days can she call
me 5 - 8 times. And we can talk
normally for a short while.
And suddenly she can ask
about something completely
different.
For example, as if the children
have come home from school.
-But they are adults, mom.
Parkinson's affect the
memory too. She can say that I
should come and pick her up,
in a place where she is not. In a
convincingly detailed manner.
But now there are many
times she says she does not
recognize herself.
In her apartment at the
nursing home. She feels unsafe.

And when she calls me early evening. I know she's not feeling well.
-Please come and help me. I don't want to be in this apartment.

I try to explain that it is her apartment she lives in.
-Look at the pictures on the wall. There are many pictures of us mom.
But it doesn't help.

My mother has been working and taken care of, accounting financial charges, all the economics stuff.

And the company did well,
so it's difficult to understand.
To get Parkinson's and a close
relationship with my mom,
it's so hard.
I want my real mother back.
Especially when she explains
the terrible pain.

Difficulty walking and falls.
Difficulty breading and
swallowing.
And her headache.
-It feels like a washing
centrifuge in my head,
she explains.
When I go to mom, I try to
give her positive energy.
But my heart aches inside.

Some people say that you
should agree, at this stage.

I have a hard time with
it, then it feels like I'm
cheating her.
But I listened to what the
others with experience said.

One afternoon when I
was there to visit.
Then I sat down on her
couch. And suddenly mom
went to get her bag.
She put down her old
mobile phone, that doesn't
work. Pictures of us in the
family. And a package of
crusts to eat.

What are you going to do
mom I asked.
-Come, we're going to my
 apartment.
-But please mom, we're in your
apartment.
-Quiet, come on and let's go.
So I followed.

We went to the elevator.
I didn't see which button
she was pressing. The elevator
started. And in the next
second, the door opened.
We were on the same floor.
And then everything was fine.

This is no longer my mother.
It's like another person.

She can also hide stuff, because
the disease symptoms can
make people paranoid.
They may believe that people
are taking their possessions.

Although it can be very
stressful and frustrating.
To see how the disease changes
a person's personality.
It is a very difficult disease to
manage.
It requires patience as a relative.

And in the midst of all
the misery.
I try to think positive thoughts.
Because my "real mother" had
joy in life, she still loves us all.

She loves her grandchildren a lot.
And helped us all, with what she
could in different ways.

Now it is our turn to take care
of her. And it feels incredibly
good that I live nearby.

After all, being able to have the
short moments with mom
feels good.

My mother has a heart of gold.
She is so caring despite her
illness.

But it is terribly hard to watch
her slowly fade away.

I know I'm not alone.
There are so many others who
have Parkinson's disease.
I hope to support someone,
with my book to feel better.
Make relatives feel that they
are not alone.
We must not feel guilty.
Together we become
strong. And other people get
important knowledge too.

This is like a family
disease in torture.
And family members may
have different opinions too.
I hope my experience help
people. It's not easy,
it's a strange and hard disease.

My mother told me a
while ago, that she wanted
to meet my father.

My dad is dead.
So in a way I understand
my mom sadly.
Now it just feels like
it's the medicine that
makes her alive.

Get medicine every two,
three hours.
It is not a worthy life.
I've told my mom that dad
is waiting for her.
She believes in it too.
And give dad a big
hug from me then I said.

**Something to reflect on,
for all people.**

*Your strength is in your
vulnerability and wisdom*

*Whatever you're
facing today.
Keep going.
Keep moving.
Keep hoping.
You can handle this.*